39 Juice Recipes That Will Quickly Reduce Constipation:

Naturally and Easily Improve Your Digestion Using Delicious and Effective Ingredients

By

Joe Correa CSN

COPYRIGHT

© 2018 Live Stronger Faster Inc.

All rights reserved

Reproduction or translation of any part of this work beyond that permitted by section 107 or 108 of the 1976 United States Copyright Act without the permission of the copyright owner is unlawful.

This publication is designed to provide accurate and authoritative information in regard to the subject matter covered. It is sold with the understanding that neither the author nor the publisher is engaged in rendering medical advice. If medical advice or assistance is needed, consult with a doctor. This book is considered a guide and should not be used in any way detrimental to your health. Consult with a physician before starting this nutritional plan to make sure it's right for you.

ACKNOWLEDGEMENTS

This book is dedicated to my friends and family that have had mild or serious illnesses so that you may find a solution and make the necessary changes in your life.

39 Juice Recipes That Will Quickly Reduce Constipation:

Naturally and Easily Improve Your Digestion Using Delicious and Effective Ingredients

By

Joe Correa CSN

CONTENTS

Copyright

Acknowledgements

About The Author

Introduction

39 Juice Recipes That Will Quickly Reduce Constipation: Naturally and Easily Improve Your Digestion Using Delicious and Effective Ingredients

Additional Titles from This Author

ABOUT THE AUTHOR

After years of Research, I honestly believe in the positive effects that proper nutrition can have over the body and mind. My knowledge and experience has helped me live healthier throughout the years and which I have shared with family and friends. The more you know about eating and drinking healthier, the sooner you will want to change your life and eating habits.

Nutrition is a key part in the process of being healthy and living longer so get started today. The first step is the most important and the most significant.

INTRODUCTION

39 Juice Recipes That Will Quickly Reduce Constipation: Naturally and Easily Improve Your Digestion Using Delicious and Effective Ingredients

By Joe Correa CSN

Most people have suffered from constipation at one point or another in their lives.

Statistically speaking, one in every 10 people, and this includes children, is regularly constipated. It is imperative to treat the root cause of constipation not only because of its dreaded physical side effects, but because the bodily waste should in fact come out of our body and should not linger on inside our system.

Some of the most common symptoms of constipation are: stomach aches, bloating, the inability to easily, regularly and completely empty bowels, loss of appetite, foul smelling stools, and general lack of well-being.

The causes of constipation are different for everyone and most are not indicative of any serious medical problems.

Some of the common causes are:

- Lack of nutrients such as fruit and vegetables which

contain fiber;
- Dehydration. It is recommended to drink eight glasses of water per day;
- Certain prescription medication such as antidepressants, diuretics, antihistamines, etc.;
- Lack of physical activity. Even thirty minutes of walking daily counts;
- Some iron and calcium supplements;
- High levels of stress

While it may be difficult to determine the exact cause of constipation in most individuals, one of the best cures is to increase your fiber intake through natural produce such as nutrient packed fruits and vegetables. Juicing is a very easy way to consume the fiber needed to reset your digestive system. Liquids, in general, are easily digestible and consuming them will allow your digestive system to rest and heal itself.

These recipes are easy to make at home and bursting with flavor and nutrients your body will crave for.

Continue drinking water while juicing, make sure you include light physical activity, such as a daily stroll outside to get some fresh air and enjoy the relief that will come to your body and soul as you repair your digestive system with these recipes.

39 JUICE RECIPES THAT WILL QUICKLY REDUCE CONSTIPATION

1. Apple Beet Juice

Ingredients:

1 small apple, cored

1 cup of beets, sliced

1 whole kiwi, sliced

¼ tsp of ceylon cinnamon, ground

Preparation:

Wash the apple and remove the core and cut into bite-sized pieces.

Wash the beets and trim off the green ends. Peel and cut into thin slices. Fill the measuring cup.

Peel the kiwi and cut lengthwise in half. Set aside.

Now process apple, beets and kiwi in a juicer until well juiced or shake.

Transfer to a serving glass and stir in the ceylon cinnamon.

Refrigerate for 15 minutes before serving.

Enjoy!

Nutritional information per serving: Kcal: 139, Protein: 3.3g, Carbs: 40.6g, Fats: 0.7g

2. Peach Plum Juice

Ingredients:

2 medium-sized peaches, pitted

2 whole plums, pitted

1 whole lemon, peeled

¼ tsp of ginger, ground

Preparation:

Wash the peaches and cut in half. Remove the pits and cut into bite-sized pieces. Set aside.

Wash the plums and cut lengthwise in half. Remove the pits and set aside.

Peel the lemons and cut lengthwise in half. Set aside.

Add ingredients into a juicer and stir thoroughly.

Transfer to a serving glass and stir in the ginger.

Nutritional information per serving: Kcal: 161, Protein: 4.2g, Carbs: 49.1g, Fats: 1.2g

3. Peach Carrots Juice

Ingredients:

2 large peaches

10 medium sized carrots

2 large sized apples

1 large sized orange, peeled

½ of a lemon, skin peeled away

Preparation:

Wash the peaches and cut in half. Remove the pits and cut into bite-sized pieces. Set aside.

Wash the carrots and peel them. Cut into small chunks and set aside.

Wash the apple and remove the core and cut into bite-sized pieces.

Peel the orange and divide into wedges. Set aside.

Peel the lemon and cut lengthwise in half. Set aside.

Add ingredients into a juicer and stir thoroughly.

Transfer to a serving glass .

Refrigerate for 15 minutes before serving.

Enjoy!

Nutritional information per serving: Kcal: 139, Protein: 3.3g, Carbs: 40.6g, Fats: 0.7g

4. Spinach Apple Green Juice

Ingredients:

1 cup of fresh spinach, chopped

1 medium-sized Granny Smith's apple, cored

1 cup of cucumber, sliced

1 small ginger knob, peeled

Preparation:

Wash the spinach thoroughly under cold running water. Slightly drain and chop into small pieces. Set aside.

Wash the apple and cut in half. Remove the core and cut into small chunks. Set aside.

Wash the cucumber and cut into thin slices. Fill the measuring cup and reserve the rest for later.

Peel the ginger and set aside.

Combine all ingredients within a juicer and enjoy this super tasty and health boosting green juice drink

Transfer to a serving glass and stir in the salt.

Serve immediately.

Nutritional information per serving: Kcal: 126, Protein: 3.6g, Carbs: 35.8g, Fats: 0.8g

5. Kiwi Mango Juice

Ingredients:

1 whole kiwi, peeled

1 cup of mango, chunked

1 cup of fresh spinach, chopped

1 small ginger knob, peeled

Preparation:

Peel the kiwi and cut lengthwise in half. Set aside.

Peel the mango and cut into small chunks. Fill the measuring cup and reserve the rest in the refrigerator.

Wash the spinach thoroughly under cold running water. Slightly drain and chop it into small pieces. Set aside.

Peel the ginger knob and set aside.

Now, combine mango, kiwi, spinach, and ginger in a juicer and process until juiced.

Transfer to a serving glass.

Refrigerate for 10 minutes before serving.

Enjoy!

Nutritional information per serving: Kcal: 190, Protein: 9.1g, Carbs: 53.6g, Fats: 2.2g

6.   Apple Avocado Asparagus Juice

Ingredients:

1 small Golden Delicious apple, cored

1 cup of avocado, cubed

1 cup of fresh asparagus, trimmed

1 whole lime, peeled

1 small ginger knob, peeled

Preparation:

Wash the apple and cut in half. Remove the core and cut into small chunks. Set aside.

Peel the avocado and cut lengthwise in half. Remove the pit and cut into small chunks. Set aside.

Wash the asparagus and trim off the woody ends. Cut into bite-sized pieces and set aside.

Peel the lime and cut lengthwise in half. Set aside.

Peel the ginger knob and cut into small pieces. Set aside.

Now, process apple, avocado, asparagus, lime and ginger in a juicer.

Transfer to a serving glass.

Refrigerate for 15 minutes before serving.

Enjoy!

Nutritional information per serving: Kcal: 298, Protein: 7.3g, Carbs: 41.6g, Fats: 22.5g

7. Mango Cantaloupe Juice

Ingredients:

1 cup of mango, chunked

1 cup of cantaloupe, diced

1 medium-sized peach, pitted

1 whole lime, peeled

¼ tsp of ceylon cinnamon, ground

Preparation:

Wash and peel the mango. Cut into small chunks and set aside.

Cut the cantaloupe in half. Scoop out the seeds and cut two wedges and peel them. Chop into chunks and set aside. Reserve the rest of the cantaloupe in a refrigerator.

Wash the peach and cut lengthwise in half. Remove the pit and cut into bite-sized pieces. Set aside.

Peel the lime and cut lengthwise in half. Set aside.

Now, combine mango, cantaloupe, peach and lime in a juicer. Process until well juiced.

Transfer to a serving glass and stir in the ceylon cinnamon.

Serve immediately.

Enjoy!

Nutritional information per serving: Kcal: 205, Protein: 5.2g, Carbs: 59.2g, Fats: 1.6g

8. Avocado Strawberry Juice

Ingredients:

1 cup of avocado, cubed

1 cup of strawberries, chopped

1 cup of cucumber, sliced

1 medium-sized orange, wedged

1 cup of Swiss chard

Preparation:

Peel the avocado and cut in half. Remove the pit and cut into cubes. Fill the measuring cup and reserve the rest for later

Wash the strawberries and cut into small pieces. Set aside.

Wash the cucumber and cut into thin slices. Fill the measuring cup and reserve the rest for later.

Peel the orange and divide into wedges. Chop each wedge in half and set aside.

Wash the Swiss chard under cold running water. Slightly drain and roughly chop it. Set aside.

Now, combine avocado, strawberries, cucumber, orange,

and Swiss chard in a juicer. Process until well juiced.

Transfer to a serving glass and add some crushed ice before serving.

Enjoy!

Nutritional information per serving: Kcal: 241, Protein: 4.24g, Carbs: 26.54g, Fats: 21.62g

9. Avocado Fennel Juice

Ingredients:

1 cup of avocado, chunked

1 cup of fennel, chopped

1 small Granny Smith's apple, chopped

1 cup of cucumber, sliced

¼ tsp of ginger, ground

Preparation:

Peel the avocado and cut in half. Remove the pit and cut into small chunks. Fill the measuring cup and reserve the rest for later.

Wash the fennel bulb and trim off the wilted outer layers. Cut into small chunks and fill the measuring cup. Reserve the rest in the refrigerator.

Wash the apple and remove the core. Cut into bite-sized pieces and set aside.

Wash the cucumber and cut into thin slices. Fill the measuring cup and reserve the rest in the refrigerator. Set aside.

Now, combine avocado, fennel, apple, and cucumber in a juicer and process until juiced.

Transfer to a serving glass and stir in the ginger.

Add some ice before serving.

Enjoy!

Nutritional information per serving: Kcal: 286, Protein: 5g, Carbs: 40.3g, Fats: 21.9g

10. Blueberry Watermelon Juice

Ingredients:

2 cups of blueberries

1 cup of watermelon, cubed

1 cup of fresh basil, torn

1 oz of water

Preparation:

Place the blueberries in a large colander. Rinse well under cold running water and set aside.

Cut one large watermelon wedge. Using a sharp paring knife, peel and cut into small cubes. Remove the seeds and set aside.

Wash the basil and roughly torn it with hands. Set aside.

Now, combine blueberries, watermelon, and basil in a juicer. Process until juiced.

Transfer to a serving glass and stir in the water.

Refrigerate for 10 minutes before serving.

Nutritional information per serving: Kcal: 188, Protein: 3.8g, Carbs: 55g, Fats: 1.3g

11. Blueberry Spinach Juice

Ingredients:

2 cups of fresh spinach, chopped

1 cup of cucumber, sliced

1 Apple, cored

1 Big Handful Blueberries

2 Carrots

¼ tsp of ginger, ground

Preparation:

Wash the spinach thoroughly under cold running water. Slightly drain and chop into small pieces. Set aside.

Wash the cucumber and cut into thin slices. Fill the measuring cup and reserve the rest for later.

Wash the apple and remove the core and cut into bite-sized pieces.

Place the blueberries in a large colander. Rinse well under cold running water and set aside.

Wash and peel the carrots. Cut into thin slices and fill the measuring cup. Reserve the rest in the refrigerator.

Now, combine spinach, cucumber, apple, blueberries and carrots in a juicer. Process until juiced.

Transfer to a serving glass and stir in the ginger.

Serve immediately.

Enjoy!

Nutritional information per serving: Kcal: 203, Protein: 4.8g, Carbs: 60.5g, Fats: 1.3g

12. Beet Orange Juice

Ingredients:

1 whole beet, sliced

1 medium-sized orange, peeled

1 cup of cucumber, sliced

1 tbsp of liquid honey

Preparation:

Wash the beet and trim off the green parts. Cut into thin slices and set aside.

Peel the orange and divide into wedges. Cut each wedge in half and set aside.

Wash the cucumber and cut into thin slices. Fill the measuring cup and reserve the rest in the refrigerator.

Now, combine beet, orange and cucumber in a juicer and process until juiced. Transfer to a serving glass and stir in the honey.

Serve immediately.

Enjoy!

Nutritional information per serving: Kcal: 83, Protein: 2.8g, Carbs: 25.1g, Fats: 0.3g

13. Green Juice

Ingredients:

4 cups of fresh spinach, chopped

4 medium green Granny Smith's apples, cored

¼ cup of fresh mint leaves, torn

3 large kale leaves, torn

3 large stalks of celery, chopped

1 ½ cup of fresh basil, torn

Preparation:

Wash the spinach thoroughly under cold running water. Chop into small pieces and fill the measuring cup. Reserve the rest for later.

Wash the apple and cut lengthwise in half. Remove the core and cut into bite-sized pieces. Set aside.

Combine kale and mint in a large colander. Wash thoroughly under cold running water. Slightly drain and torn with hands. Set aside.

Wash the celery stalk and cut into small pieces. Set aside.

Wash the basil and roughly torn it with hands. Set aside.

Place all ingredients through a juicer and blend together. Process until juiced.

Refrigerate for 10 minutes before serving.

Enjoy!

Nutritional information per serving: Kcal: 425, Protein: 17.2g, Carbs: 122.2g Fats: 4.1g

14. Carrot Plum Juice

Ingredients:

4 whole plum, chopped

1 cup of carrots, sliced

1 cup of Romaine lettuce, shredded

1 cup of mustard greens, torn

1 oz of water

Preparation:

Wash the plums and cut each in half. Remove the pits and set aside.

Wash and peel the carrots. Cut into thin slices and fill the measuring cup. Reserve the rest in the refrigerator.

Combine lettuce and mustard greens in a large colander. Rinse well under cold running water. Shred the lettuce torn the mustard greens using hands. Set aside.

Now, combine carrots, plums, lettuce, and mustard greens in a juicer and process until juiced. Transfer to a serving glass and stir in the water.

Serve cold.

Nutritional information per serving: Kcal: 128, Protein: 4.8g, Carbs: 39.1g, Fats: 1.3g

15. Avocado Raspberry Juice

Ingredients:

1 cup of avocado, chunked

1 cup of raspberries

1 small peach, pitted

3 whole apricots, chopped

¼ tsp of ceylon cinnamon, ground

Preparation:

Peel the avocado and cut lengthwise in half. Cut into thin slices and reserve the rest in the refrigerator. Set aside.

Wash the raspberries using a colander. Slightly drain and fill the measuring cup. Reserve the rest in the refrigerator or freezer for later.

Wash the peach and cut in half. Remove the pit and cut into bite-sized pieces. Set aside.

Wash the apricots and cut in half. Remove the pits and cut in quarters. Set aside.

Now, combine avocado, raspberries, peach, and apricots in a juicer and process until juiced.

Transfer to a serving glass and stir in the ceylon cinnamon.

Refrigerate for 15 minutes before serving.

Enjoy!

Nutritional information per serving: Kcal: 206, Protein: 5.5g, Carbs: 63.5g, Fats: 2.1g

16. Celery Kale Juice

Ingredients:

2 medium-sized celery stalk, chopped

1 cup of fresh kale, chopped

1 small apple, cored

1 cup of Romaine lettuce, shredded

1 ½ cup of fresh basil, torn

Preparation:

Wash the celery stalks and cut into bite-sized pieces. Set aside

Wash the kale thoroughly under cold running water. Slightly drain and chop it into small pieces. Set aside.

Wash the apple and cut in half. Remove the core and cut into small pieces. Set aside.

Wash the lettuce leaves and shred it. Fill the measuring cup and reserve the rest for later.

Wash the basil and roughly torn it with hands. Set aside.

Now, combine kale, celery, apple, lettuce and basil in a juicer and process until juiced.

Transfer to a serving glass and add some ice before serving.

Enjoy!

Nutritional information per serving: Kcal: 103, Protein: 4.6g, Carbs: 29.4g, Fats: 1.2g

17. Spinach Cauliflower Juice

Ingredients:

2 cup of fresh spinach, torn

5 cauliflower flowerets, chopped

2 cup of black grapes

1 oz of water

¼ tsp of ginger, ground

Preparation:

Wash the spinach thoroughly under running water. Torn with hands and set aside.

Wash the cauliflower flowerets and chop into small pieces. Fill the measuring cup and reserve the rest for later.

Wash the grapes and fill the measuring cup. Reserve the rest for later.

Now, combine cauliflower, spinach and grapes in a juicer and process until juiced.

Transfer to a serving glass and stir in the water and ginger.

Add some ice and serve immediately.

Enjoy!

Nutritional information per serving: Kcal: 136, Protein: 4.1g, Carbs: 36.9g, Fats: 1g

18. Grape Blueberry Juice

Ingredients:

1 cup of black grapes

1 cup of blueberries

1 small Golden Delicious apple, cored

¼ tsp of cinnamon, ground

Preparation:

Wash the grapes and fill the measuring cup. Reserve the rest for later.

Wash the blueberries using a colander. Slightly drain and set aside.

Wash the apple and cut in half. Remove the core and cut into bite-sized pieces. Set aside.

Now, combine grapes, blueberries and apple in a juicer and process until juiced.

Transfer to a serving glass and stir in the cinnamon.

Add some ice before serving.

Enjoy!

Nutritional information per serving: Kcal: 191, Protein: 2.1g, Carbs: 54.7g, Fats: 1g

19. Blueberry Grapes Juice

Ingredients:

2 cups of blueberries

1 cup of black grapes

1 medium-sized blood orange, peeled

1 small ginger knob, peeled and chopped

Preparation:

Place the blueberries in a colander. Wash thoroughly under cold running water and drain. Fill the measuring cups and reserve the rest in the freezer.

Wash the grapes and fill the measuring cup. Set aside.

Peel the orange and divide into wedges. Cut each wedge in half and set aside.

Peel the ginger and cut into small pieces. Set aside.

Now, combine blueberries, grapes, orange and ginger in a juicer and process until juiced.

Transfer to a serving glass and add few ice cubes before serving.

Enjoy!

Nutritional information per serving: Kcal: 254, Protein: 4.1g, Carbs: 75.2g, Fats: 1.5g

20. Kiwi Broccoli Juice

Ingredients:

1 whole kiwi, sliced

1 cup of broccoli, chopped

1 medium-sized Granny Smith's apple, cored

1 medium-sized celery stalk, cut into bite-sized pieces

1 cup of fresh spinach, chopped

1 small ginger knob, peeled and chopped

Preparation:

Peel the kiwi and cut lengthwise in half. Set aside.

Wash the broccoli and chop into small pieces. Set aside.

Wash the apple and cut in half. Remove the core and cut into small chunks. Set aside.

Wash the celery and cut into bite-sized pieces. Set aside.

Wash the spinach thoroughly under cold running water. Chop into small pieces and fill the measuring cup. Reserve the rest for later.

Peel the ginger knob and chop it into small pieces. Set

aside.

Now, combine kiwi, broccoli, apple, celery, spinach and ginger in a juicer and process until well juiced.

Transfer to serving glass and add some ice before serving.

Enjoy!

Nutritional information per serving: Kcal: 146, Protein: 1.2g, Carbs: 42.2g, Fats: 1.2g

21. Artichoke Spinach Juice

Ingredients:

1 medium-sized artichoke, chopped

1 cup of fresh spinach, chopped

2 cup of black grapes

1 Big Handful Blueberries

1 small ginger knob, peeled and sliced

Preparation:

Trim off the outer leaves of the artichoke using a sharp paring knife. Wash it and cut into bite-sized pieces. Set aside.

Using a colander, rinse the spinach thoroughly under cold running water. Chop into small pieces and set aside.

Wash the grapes and fill the measuring cup. Reserve the rest for later.

Place the blueberries in a large colander. Rinse well under cold running water and set aside.

Peel the ginger knob and chop it into small pieces. Set aside.

Now, combine artichoke, spinach, black grapes, blueberries and ginger in a juicer and process until juiced.

Transfer to a serving glass and refrigerate for 10 minutes before serving.

Enjoy!

Nutritional information per serving: Kcal: 229, Protein: 7.4g, Carbs: 68.6g, Fats: 1.4g

22. Cabbage Avocado Juice

Ingredients:

1 cup of avocado, sliced

1 cup of purple cabbage, chopped

1 whole leek, chopped

1 medium-sized pear, chopped

½ lime, peeled

Preparation:

Peel the avocado and cut lengthwise in half. Cut into thin slices and reserve the rest in the refrigerator. Set aside.

Wash the cabbage thoroughly and chop into small pieces. Set aside.

Wash the leek and cut into bite-sized pieces. Set aside.

Wash the pear and remove the core. Cut into bite-sized pieces and set aside.

Peel the lime and cut lengthwise in half. Set aside.

Now, combine avocado, cabbage, leek, pear and lime in a juicer and process until juiced.

Transfer to a serving glass and refrigerate for 15 minutes before serving.

Enjoy!

Nutritional information per serving: Kcal: 352, Protein: 6.35g, Carbs: 62.41g, Fats: 22.09g

23. Red Juice

Ingredients:

2 leaves of purple cabbage, chopped

2 medium-sized Red Delicious apple, cored

3 medium-sized carrot, sliced

1 cup of strawberries, sliced

¼ beet, sliced

Preparation:

Wash the cabbage thoroughly and chop into small pieces. Set aside.

Wash the apple and cut in half. Remove the core and cut into small chunks. Set aside.

Wash and peel carrots. Cut into thin slices and set aside.

Wash the strawberries and remove the stems. Cut into small pieces and fill the measuring cup. Set aside.

Wash the beets and trim off the green parts. Cut into bite-sized pieces and set aside.

Now, combine cabbage, apple, carrot, strawberries and beet in a juicer and process until juiced.

Transfer to a serving glass and refrigerate for 10 minutes before serving.

Enjoy!

Nutritional information per serving: Kcal: 302, Protein: 5.2g, Carbs: 88.6g, Fats: 1.4g

24. Cauliflower Beet greens Juice

Ingredients:

1 cup of cauliflower, chopped

1 cup of beet greens, torn

1 cup of fresh basil, torn

1 medium-sized red apple, cored

1 large lemon, peeled

1 cup of broccoli, chopped

Preparation:

Trim off the outer leaves of a cauliflower. Wash it and fill and cut into small pieces. Fill the measuring cup and reserve the rest in the refrigerator.

Combine beet greens and basil in a large colander. Rinse under cold running water and drain. Torn with hands and set aside.

Wash the apple and cut lengthwise in half. Remove the core and cut into bite-sized pieces. Set aside.

Peel the lemon and cut lengthwise in half. Set aside.

Wash the broccoli and chop into small pieces. Set aside.

Now, combine cauliflower, beet greens, basil, apple, lemon and broccoli, in a juicer. Process until well juiced and transfer to a serving glass.

Add few ice cubes and serve immediately.

Enjoy!

Nutritional information per serving: Kcal: 137, Protein: 7.3g, Carbs: 42.1g, Fats: 1.3g

25. Beet Orange Juice

Ingredients:

2 large beets, trimmed and chopped

1 large orange, wedged

1 cup of broccoli, chopped

1 large cucumber, sliced

Preparation:

Wash the beets and trim off the green parts. Cut into bite-sized pieces and set aside.

Peel the orange and divide into wedges. Set aside.

Wash the broccoli and cut into bite-sized pieces. Fill the measuring cup and reserve the rest for later.

Wash the cucumber and cut into thin slices. Set aside.

Now, combine beets, orange, broccoli, and cucumber in a juicer and process until juiced.

Garnish with some fresh mint, if you like.

Transfer to a serving glass and add some ice before serving.

Enjoy!

Nutritional information per serving: Kcal: 123, Protein: 7.8g, Carbs: 38.1g, Fats: 1.1g

26. Cauliflower Kale Juice

Ingredients:

1 cup of cauliflower, chopped

1 cup of fresh kale, torn

1 cup of broccoli, chopped

1 small green apple, cored

¼ teaspoon of ginger, ground

Preparation:

Wash the cauliflower and trim off the outer leaves. Cut into small pieces and set aside.

Rinse the kale under cold running water and slightly drain. Torn with hands and set aside.

Wash the broccoli thoroughly and chop into small pieces. Set aside.

Wash the apple and cut lengthwise in half. remove the core and cut into bite-sized pieces. Set aside.

Now, combine cauliflower, kale, broccoli, cauliflower, apple and kale in a juicer and process until well juiced.

Transfer to a serving glass and stir in the ground ginger.

Enjoy!

Nutritional information per serving: Kcal: 131, Protein: 8.1g, Carbs: 36.8g, Fats: 1.5g

27. Broccoli Grapes Juice

Ingredients:

1 cup of fresh broccoli, chopped

1 cup of green grapes

1 cup of cucumber, sliced

1 cup of mustard greens, torn

1 small ginger knob, peeled

2 oz of water

Preparation:

Wash the broccoli and cut into bite-sized pieces. Set aside.

Wash the grapes and set aside.

Wash the cucumber and cut into thin slices. Fill the measuring cup and reserve the rest for later.

Rinse the mustard greens thoroughly under cold running water. Torn with hands and set aside.

Peel the ginger knob and set aside.

Now, combine broccoli, grapes, cucumber, mustard greens and ginger in a juicer and process until juiced.

Transfer to a serving glass and stir in the water.

Add some ice and serve immediately.

Enjoy!

Nutritional information per serving: Kcal: 100, Protein: 5.2g, Carbs: 27.4g, Fats: 1g

28. Grape Watermelon Juice

Ingredients:

1 cup of green grapes

1 cup of watermelon, cubed

1 whole kiwi, peeled

1 medium-sized pear, chopped

¼ tsp of ceylon cinnamon, ground

Preparation:

Wash the grapes and set aside.

Cut the watermelon lengthwise. Cut one large wedge and peel it. Cut into chunks and fill the measuring cup. Remove the seeds and set aside. Reserve the rest of the melon for some other juices.

Peel the kiwi and cut lengthwise in half. Set aside.

Wash the pear and remove the core. Cut into bite-sized pieces and set aside.

Now, combine watermelon, grapes, kiwi, and pear in a juicer and process until well juiced.

Transfer to a serving glass and stir in the ceylon cinnamon

Enjoy!

Nutritional information per serving: Kcal: 216, Protein: 3g, Carbs: 64.5g, Fats: 1.2g

29. Cabbage Kale Kiwi Juice

Ingredients:

1 cup of cabbage, shredded

1 cup of fresh kale, torn

2 cups of fresh spinach, torn

1 cup of fresh parsley, torn

1 cup of cucumber, sliced

1 whole kiwi, peeled

1 cup of avocado, chunked

¼ tsp of turmeric, ground

Preparation:

Wash the cabbage thoroughly and shred the cabbage. Fill the measuring cup and reserve the rest for later.

Combine kale, spinach and parsley in a large colander. Rinse all under cold running water and slightly drain. Torn with hands and set aside.

Wash the cucumber and cut into thin slices. Set aside.

Peel the kiwi and cut lengthwise in half. Set aside

Peel the avocado and cut in half. Remove the pit and cut into small chunks. Fill the measuring cup and reserve the rest for later.

Now, combine cabbage, kale, spinach, parsley, cucumber, kiwi and avocado in a juicer and process until juiced.

Transfer to a serving glass and stir in the turmeric.

Refrigerate for 10 minutes and serve.

Enjoy!

Nutritional information per serving: Kcal: 290, Protein: 10.7g, Carbs: 40.3g, Fats: 23.1g

30. Orange Beet Juice

Ingredients:

1 small blood orange, wedged

1 cup of beets, trimmed and sliced

1 cup of avocado, cubed

½ cup of green grapes

Preparation:

Peel the orange and divide into wedges. Cut each wedge in half and set aside.

Wash the beets thoroughly and trim off the green parts, Cut into thin slices and fill the measuring cup. Reserve the rest in the refrigerator. .

Peel the avocado and cut lengthwise in half. Cut into small cubes and fill the measuring cup. Reserve the rest for later.

Wash the grapes and fill the measuring cup. Set aside.

Now, combine orange, beets, avocado, and grapes in a juicer. Add few ice cubes and process until juiced.

Garnish with some fresh mint, if you like

Transfer to a serving glass and serve immediately.

Enjoy!

Nutrition information per serving: Kcal: 350, Protein: 7.3g, Carbs: 56.1g, Fats: 22.6g

31. Grapes Cherry Juice

Ingredients:

1 cup of black grapes

1 cup of cherries, pitted

1 cup of blueberries

1 small blood orange, wedged

¼ tsp of cinnamon, ground

Preparation:

Wash the cherries and cut each in half. Remove the pits and set aside.

Combine blueberries and grapes in a colander and wash under cold running water. Slightly drain and set aside.

Peel the orange and divide into wedges. Cut each wedge in half and set aside.

Now, combine grapes, blueberries, cherries and orange in a juicer and process until juiced.

Transfer to a serving glass and stir in the cinnamon.

Add some ice and serve immediately.

Enjoy!

Nutritional information per serving: Kcal: 249, Protein: 4.2g, Carbs: 73.2g, Fats: 1.2g

32.   Avocado Broccoli Juice

Ingredients:

1 cup of avocado, cubed

1 cup of broccoli, chopped

1 medium-sized orange, peeled

1 cup of fresh kale, torn

2 large kiwis, peeled

Preparation:

Peel the avocado cut lengthwise in half. Remove the pit and cut into small cubes. Fill the measuring cup and reserve the rest for later. Set aside.

Wash the broccoli and cut into small pieces. Set aside.

Peel the orange and divide into wedges. Set aside.

Rinse the kale under cold running water and slightly drain. Torn with hands and set aside.

Peel the kiwis and cut lengthwise in half. Set aside.

Now, combine avocado, broccoli, orange, kale and kiwis under seeds in a juicer and process until juiced.

Transfer to a serving glass and add some ice before serving.

Garnish with some fresh mint, if you like. However, it's optional.

Enjoy!

Nutrition information per serving: Kcal: 357, Protein: 11.1g, Carbs: 59.9g, Fats: 23.2g

33. Spinach Kiwi Juice

Ingredients:

1 cup of fresh spinach, torn

¼ cup of fresh mint leaves

2 whole kiwis, peeled

1 small apple, cored

1 small peach, pitted

Preparation:

Rinse the spinach under cold running water and slightly drain. Torn with hands and set aside.

Combine spinach and mint in a large colander. Wash thoroughly under cold running water. Slightly drain and torn with hands. Set aside.

Peel the kiwis and cut lengthwise in half. Set aside.

Wash the apple and cut in half. Remove the core and cut into bite-sized pieces. Set aside.

Wash the peach and cut in half. Remove the pit and cut into bite-sized pieces. Set aside.

Now, combine spinach, kiwis, apple and peach in a juicer

and process until juiced. Transfer to a serving glass and add some ice.

Serve immediately.

Enjoy!

Nutrition information per serving: Kcal: 199, Protein: 5.3g, Carbs: 58.9g, Fats: 1.7g

34. Orange Blackberry Juice

Ingredients:

1 medium-sized orange, peeled

1 cup of blackberries

1 cup of watermelon, cubed

1 tbsp of liquid honey

¼ tsp of cinnamon, ground

Preparation:

Peel the orange and divide into wedges. Cut each wedge in half and set aside.

Wash the blackberries thoroughly under cold water and slightly drain. Set aside.

Cut the watermelon in half. Cut one large wedge and wrap the rest in a plastic foil and refrigerate. Peel the slice and cut into small cubes. Remove the pits and fill the measuring cup. Set aside.

Wash the blackberries thoroughly under cold water and slightly drain. Set aside.

Now, combine watermelon, blackberries, and orange in a

juicer and process until juiced. Transfer to a serving glass and stir in the honey and cinnamon.

Refrigerate for 10 minutes before serving.

Enjoy!

Nutrition information per serving: Kcal: 186, Protein: 4.2g, Carbs: 40.7g, Fats: 1.1g

35. Apples Grapes Green Juice

Ingredients:

2 medium sized Granny Smith apples, cored

1 cup of cucumber, sliced

17 green grapes

2 cup of fresh spinach, torn

Preparation:

Wash the apple and cut in half. Remove the core and cut into bite-sized pieces. Set aside.

Wash the cucumber and cut into thin slices. Fill the measuring cup and reserve the rest for later.

Wash the grapes and fill the measuring cup. Set aside.

Wash the spinach thoroughly and slightly drain. Torn with hands and set aside.

Now, combine apple, cucumber, grapes and spinach in a juicer and process until juiced.

Transfer to a serving glass . Garnish with some fresh mint, if you like. However, it's optional.

Enjoy!

Nutrition information per serving: Kcal: 127, Protein: 3.13g, Carbs: 33.77g, Fats: 0.79g

36. Strawberry Mango Juice

Ingredients:

½ cup of strawberries, cut into bite-sized pieces

1 cup of mango, chunked

1 small apple, cored

2 whole cherries, pitted

1 tsp of dried mint, ground

Preparation:

Wash the strawberries and remove the core. Cut into bite-sized pieces and set aside.

Peel the mango and cut into bite-sized pieces. Set aside.

Wash the apple and cut in half. Remove the core and cut into small pieces. Set aside.

Wash the cherries and cut each in half. Remove the pits and set aside.

Place the mint in a small bowl and add two tablespoons of hot water. Let it soak for 5 minutes.

Now, combine mango, strawberries, apple, cherries and mint mixture in a juicer and process until juiced. Transfer to a serving glass and refrigerate for 15 minutes before serving.

Enjoy!

Nutritional information per serving: Kcal: 185, Protein: 2.8g, Carbs: 53.8g, Fats: 1.1g

37. Kale Broccoli Juice

Ingredients:

2 cups of kale, roughly chopped

2 cups of broccoli, chopped

2 medium-sized asparagus spears, trimmed

1 cup of fresh mint, torn

1 whole lemon, peeled

1 small ginger knob, peeled

Preparation:

Rinse the kale under cold running water. Slightly drain and torn with hands. Set aside.

Trim off the outer leaves of the broccoli. Wash it and cut into bite-sized pieces. Set aside.

Wash the asparagus and trim off the woody ends. Cut into small pieces and set aside.

Wash the mint and roughly chop it. You can soak it in water for 5 minutes before preparation, but it's optional. Set aside.

Peel the ginger knob and set aside.

Peel the lemon and cut lengthwise in half. Set aside.

Now, combine broccoli, kale, asparagus, ginger, mint, and lemon in a juicer. Process until juiced. Transfer to a serving glass and refrigerate for 15 minutes before serving.

Enjoy!

Nutritional information per serving: Kcal: 118, Protein: 13.3g, Carbs: 35.3g, Fats: 2.4g

38. Apple Celery Juice

Ingredients:

1 large green apple, cored

1 large lemon, peeled

3 large celery stalks, chopped

1 large cucumber

2 oz of coconut water

Preparation:

Wash the apple and cut lengthwise in half. Remove the core and cut into small chunks. Set aside.

Peel the lemon and cut lengthwise in half. Set aside.

Wash the celery stalks and cut into small pieces. Set aside.

Peel the cucumber and cut into small chunks. Set aside.

Now, combine apple, lemon, celery, and cucumber in a juicer and process until well juiced. Transfer to serving glasses and stir in the coconut water.

Add few ice cubes and serve immediately.

Enjoy!

Nutritional information per serving: Kcal: 175, Protein: 5.1g, Carbs: 50.2g, Fats: 1.3g

39. Kale Carrot Juice

Ingredients:

1 cup of fresh kale, chopped

1 large carrot, sliced

1 large celery, chopped

1 small Granny Smith's apple, cored

1 tbsp of liquid honey

Preparation:

Rinse the kale under cold running water using a colander. Slightly drain and torn with hands. Set aside.

Wash and peel the carrot. Cut into thin slices and set aside.

Wash the celery and cut into bite-sized pieces. Set aside.

Wash the apple and cut lengthwise in half. Remove the core and cut into bite-sized pieces. Set aside.

Now, combine kale, carrot, celery, and apple in a juicer and process until juiced. Transfer to a serving glass and stir in the honey.

Add some ice and serve immediately.

Enjoy!

Nutritional information per serving: Kcal: 179, Protein: 4.6g, Carbs: 34.3g, Fats: 1.1g

ADDITIONAL TITLES FROM THIS AUTHOR

70 Effective Meal Recipes to Prevent and Solve Being Overweight: Burn Fat Fast by Using Proper Dieting and Smart Nutrition

By

Joe Correa CSN

48 Acne Solving Meal Recipes: The Fast and Natural Path to Fixing Your Acne Problems in Less Than 10 Days!

By

Joe Correa CSN

41 Alzheimer's Preventing Meal Recipes: Reduce or Eliminate Your Alzheimer's Condition in 30 Days or Less!

By

Joe Correa CSN

70 Effective Breast Cancer Meal Recipes: Prevent and Fight Breast Cancer with Smart Nutrition and Powerful Foods

By

Joe Correa CSN

www.ingramcontent.com/pod-product-compliance
Lightning Source LLC
Chambersburg PA
CBHW030301030426
42336CB00009B/472